BODY CONTOURING TECHNIQUES FOR BEGINNERS

Sculpting, Shaping, And Toning Methods For Effective Fat Reduction And Muscle Definition

DR SAWYER DIEGO

DISCLAMER

Nothing in this book should be interpreted as medical advice; it is meant exclusively for educational reasons. Regarding their specific health issues and treatment options, readers are urged to speak with licensed healthcare professionals. The publisher and author disclaim all liability for any errors or omissions in the material provided, as well as for any negative effects that may arise from using or abusing the information. Although every attempt has been taken to guarantee that the material in this book is correct as of the date of publishing, new research may have superseded some of the content because medical knowledge is always changing. It is recommended that readers confirm the most recent medical recommendations and guidelines. The reader of this book undertakes to release the author and publisher from any claims or liabilities resulting from the use of this information, and understands and accepts the inherent risks connected with healthcare decisions.

TABLE OF CONTENTS

ABOUT THE BOOK

Body contouring includes both surgical and non-surgical methods intended to sculpt and enhance body contours, addressing areas of concern such as stubborn fat deposits or loose skin. "Body Contouring Techniques for Beginners" is a comprehensive guide for individuals exploring body contouring procedures, to educate and inform readers about the various techniques, considerations, and expectations associated with reshaping the body.

By outlining the advantages of these procedures, the book explains how body contouring can assist people in achieving their desired aesthetic goals, whether through liposuction or non-invasive procedures like CoolSculpting and laser therapy.

It highlights the importance of selecting procedures that are tailored to individual needs, supported by a thorough understanding of basic anatomy and the physiological processes involved. Grasping the transformative impact of body contouring on one's physical appearance and confidence is the first step towards appreciating its significance.

A crucial topic addressed in the book is safety and hygiene procedures, so readers will know how important it is to choose licensed providers and facilities. It also explores pre-procedure planning, which includes consultation procedures, patient eligibility evaluations, and the psychological aspects that are critical for controlling expectations and guaranteeing a good experience.

Comprehensive chapters delve deeper into particular techniques, such as the differences between modern and traditional liposuction techniques, anesthetic options, and the subtle steps involved in each procedure; they also provide insight into non-surgical options, their mechanisms of action, and combination strategies that can improve their efficacy for a variety of body types.

The book also covers potential risks and complications related to body contouring, providing readers with knowledge on minimizing these risks and understanding their responsibilities during the recovery phase. Post-procedure care and recovery are extensively discussed, offering helpful advice on managing discomfort, adhering to appropriate diet and nutrition guidelines, and maintaining long-term results.

The value proposition of various procedures, financing options, and cost factors are all included. Readers are guided through the process of choosing the best clinic and provider, with a focus on the significance of facility standards, patient testimonials, and research to make well-informed decisions.

Anticipating technological breakthroughs, patient preferences, and external factors that could impact the industry, the book looks ahead to explore future trends in body contouring. A dedicated FAQ section clarifies frequently asked questions regarding recovery times, procedure combinations, and long-term results.

"Body Contouring Techniques for Beginners" is an essential tool for people who are just starting in the body contouring industry. It provides them with the information, perspectives, and hands-on coaching they need to confidently and sensibly traverse this revolutionary area.

CHAPTER ONE

BODY CONTOURING TECHNIQUES OVERVIEW

BODY CONTOURING: WHAT IS IT?

Body contouring is the term for a group of aesthetic procedures used to improve the overall shape and proportions of the body by tightening loose skin, sculpting specific areas, and reducing excess fat. Common procedures include body lifts, liposuction, tummy tucks, and non-invasive treatments like ultrasound fat reduction and laser therapy.

The main objective of body contouring is to make the body look more attractive by focusing on areas that might not respond well to diet and exercise alone. This is a very individualized process, with treatment plans made specifically for each patient's anatomy and desired results. Experts in this field use cutting-edge techniques to produce results that are natural-looking while minimizing patient discomfort and recovery time.

hen it comes to body contouring, it is important to understand the fundamentals of the procedure. First and foremost, whether one is dealing with localized fat deposits or sagging skin following weight loss, effective body contouring necessitates a comprehensive approach that takes into account both the physical and psychological aspects of transformation.

Practitioners use state-of-the-art technologies and customized treatment plans to improve body confidence and overall well-being.

ADVANTAGES OF TECHNIQUES FOR BODY CONTOURING

Beyond cosmetic enhancement, body contouring techniques offer many advantages. By addressing areas of concern that may have been difficult to improve through diet and exercise alone, these procedures often boost confidence and self-esteem in their patients. By tightening skin and removing excess fat, body contouring can create a more toned and youthful appearance, which in turn helps patients feel more comfortable and satisfied with their bodies.

In addition, body contouring has benefits beyond appearances. Reducing fat in particular areas can ease the strain on joints and muscles, which may improve mobility and lessen the discomfort associated with being overweight.

These procedures can also improve overall comfort and quality of life by tightening loose skin and preventing chafing and irritation.

The psychological benefits of body contouring are substantial, and after the procedure, many patients report feeling more driven to continue living a healthy lifestyle, which leads to long-lasting improvements in eating and exercise habits. This positive reinforcement loop promotes long-term well-being and helps people maintain their desired body shape over time.

ANATOMY AND PHYSIOLOGY FUNDAMENTALS RELATED TO BODY CONTOURING

Successful body contouring procedures require a basic understanding of anatomy and physiology. Practitioners need to be well-versed in the body's musculoskeletal structure, patterns of fat distribution, and skin elasticity to plan and carry out treatments effectively. Depending on the patient's goals and the unique anatomical characteristics of each area of the body, different approaches may be needed.

For example, to achieve a flatter, more defined abdomen, abdominal contouring procedures frequently target the rectus abdominis muscles and the superficial fascia layer. It is also critical for practitioners to understand the vascular and lymphatic systems to reduce the risk of complications, such as bruising, swelling, or impaired healing.

By doing so, they can tailor treatment plans that maximize results while putting patient safety and comfort first.

In addition, understanding skin physiology is essential to selecting the right methods for skin tightening and rejuvenation. Elements like collagen synthesis, skin elasticity, and thickness impact the selection of procedures, whether they are non-invasive or surgical. By fusing cutting-edge technological advancements with anatomical knowledge, professionals can provide customized solutions that meet the specific anatomical and aesthetic objectives of each patient.

OVERVIEW OF TOOLS AND EQUIPMENT

Advanced imaging technologies, such as ultrasound and laser devices, facilitate the precise targeting of fat deposits while minimizing damage to surrounding tissues. Surgical instruments, such as liposuction cannulas and tissue-dissecting tools, are used to remove excess fat and sculpt specific areas of the body. A variety of specialized tools and equipment are needed for body contouring procedures to improve precision, safety, and patient comfort.

To destroy fat cells selectively without affecting nearby structures, non-invasive techniques frequently make use of devices that deliver controlled cooling, heat, or ultrasound energy.

Examples of these devices are radiofrequency machines, cryolipolysis machines, and high-intensity focused ultrasound (HIFU) systems. Each tool has a specific function in achieving desired body contours and comes in varying degrees of invasiveness and downtime.

High-quality surgical suites or treatment rooms are equipped with advanced monitoring systems, sterile draping materials, and ergonomic patient positioning devices to optimize surgical outcomes and minimize complications. Comprehensive training in equipment operation and maintenance is essential for ensuring procedural excellence and patient satisfaction.

In addition to procedural tools, equipment for patient monitoring and anesthesia administration ensures safety throughout the treatment process.

SAFETY MEASURES AND PERSONAL HYGIENE

To prevent infections, minimize risks, and promote the best possible healing outcome, it is essential to maintain strict safety precautions and hygiene practices during body contouring procedures. Sterile techniques, such as proper hand hygiene, sterile draping of surgical sites, and disinfection of equipment and instruments, are strictly adhered to in both surgical and non-surgical settings.

A thorough recovery and a lower risk of complications are supported by pre-procedural assessments, which include patient medical histories and physical examinations; these aid in identifying any contraindications or underlying health issues that may affect treatment outcomes; and they also facilitate clear communication with patients regarding post-operative care instructions, which include wound care, activity restrictions, and medication management.

Additionally, keeping the clinical space tidy and orderly promotes a culture of professionalism and safety. Consistent equipment upkeep, calibration checks, and adherence to infection control protocols guarantee regulatory compliance and encourage patient trust in the caliber of care received. By putting safety first throughout the entire treatment process, professionals uphold ethical standards and improve patient satisfaction with their body contouring experience.

CHAPTER TWO

BODY CONTOURING PROCEDURE TYPES

TECHNIQUES AND VARIATIONS FOR LIPOSUCTION

While there are differences in technique, the basic objective of body contouring procedures such as liposuction remains the same: to sculpt and reshape specific areas of the body. For example, traditional liposuction involves making small incisions near the treatment area through which a thin tube (cannula) is inserted to suction out excess fat, allowing for precise contouring of areas like the chin, arms, legs, and abdomen. More advanced techniques, like tumescent liposuction, involve injecting a saline solution mixed with an anesthetic to minimize bleeding and discomfort, improving safety and recovery.

Ultrasound-assisted liposuction (UAL) is another technique that is becoming more and more popular. It works especially well in fibrous areas like the upper back or male breast tissue. Similarly, laser-assisted liposuction (LAL) uses laser energy to liquefy fat cells, making them easier to remove. The results of both techniques are often smoother skin and shorter recovery times than with traditional methods. The surgeon's experience, the patient's anatomy, and the desired outcomes all play a role in ensuring customized outcomes that satisfy each patient's aesthetic goals.

Post-procedure care includes monitoring for any signs of infection, adhering to prescribed medications, and attending follow-up appointments to assess progress and ensure optimal healing. People who are knowledgeable about the subtleties of each liposuction technique are better able to make decisions about body contouring, which improves confidence and overall well-being. Following liposuction, patients are typically advised to wear compression garments to reduce swelling and support the newly contoured areas.

NON-SURGICAL OPTIONS: LASER THERAPY, ULTRASOUND, AND COOLSCULPTING

Non-surgical options such as CoolSculpting, ultrasound, and laser therapy are good substitutes for surgery for those seeking body contouring. CoolSculpting, also known as cryolipolysis, is a non-invasive procedure that targets stubborn fat pockets in areas like the abdomen, flanks, and thighs without damaging surrounding tissues. The body naturally eliminates the treated fat cells over weeks, leading to a gradual but noticeable reduction in fat and improved body contours.

Particularly useful for tightening and toning loose skin, ultrasound therapy (Ultherapy, etc.) uses focused ultrasound waves to penetrate deep into the skin and target underlying fat deposits. The heat energy heats and disrupts fat cells, which are then metabolized and eliminated by the body's natural processes. Laser therapy (SculpSure, etc.) uses heat energy to target fat cells selectively while protecting the skin's surface. This minimally invasive method can treat multiple areas in a single session.

Knowing the advantages and disadvantages of each non-surgical option enables people to make an informed decision about which non-surgical method is best for them. With minimal downtime compared to surgical procedures, these non-surgical techniques offer customized treatments tailored to individual needs. Patients can usually resume normal activities immediately after sessions, and they will see gradual improvements over several weeks as their bodies naturally eliminate treated fat cells.

TARGET BODY CONTOURING AREAS

Body contouring is a technique that targets specific areas where loose skin or localized fat deposits detract from desired aesthetic proportions. Common target areas include the arms; buttocks, abdomen, and chin, where fat tends to accumulate despite efforts to maintain a healthy diet and exercise regimen.

Each area has its own set of unique challenges and considerations that must be taken into account to achieve effective treatment. For example, liposuction or non-surgical techniques like CoolSculpting may be necessary to sculpt and define the waistline in the abdomen, while ultrasound therapy may be beneficial to smooth cellulite and reduce fat deposits in the thighs.

Understanding which areas can be effectively targeted with different body contouring procedures allows individuals to achieve balanced, harmonious results tailored to their unique anatomy and aesthetic goals. The buttocks, which are often a focal point for enhancement, can be contoured with procedures like Brazilian butt lift (BBL) to augment volume using a patient's fat or fillers. The arms, which are prone to sagging skin and excess fat, may undergo liposuction or skin tightening treatments to restore youthful contours and firmness.

TAILORING PROCESSES TO SPECIFIC REQUIREMENTS

Whether a patient chooses non-surgical or surgical methods, the secret to successful body contouring is to customize procedures to meet specific needs and goals. This way, doctors can recommend techniques and approaches that best suit the patient's anatomy and maximize aesthetic results while minimizing risks and complications associated with one-size-fits-all treatments. Surgeons evaluate factors like skin elasticity, fat distribution, and overall body proportions to ensure that patients achieve desired outcomes while maintaining natural-looking results.

Customization starts with a thorough consultation in which patients talk to their provider about their expectations, concerns, and medical history. Surgeons then work with patients to develop a customized treatment plan that may involve several techniques or a phased approach to achieve gradual improvements. For instance, combining radiofrequency or ultrasound therapy with liposuction to address skin laxity and reduce fat can maximize contouring results while addressing both areas of skin laxity and fat reduction. Strategic combinations of non-surgical options can also improve overall body contours without invasive surgery.

By customizing procedures to each patient's needs, providers guarantee that their enhancements will look natural and complement their body shapes and lifestyles. Follow-up visits allow for necessary adjustments, guaranteeing long-term satisfaction and confidence in the results.

EXPECTATIONS FOR RECUPERATION AND AFTER-PROCEDURE CARE

Successful body contouring outcomes depend on controlling recovery expectations and following post-procedure care instructions. Whether a patient has non-surgical or surgical procedures, knowing when to recover and how to properly care for treated areas will promote healing and maximize results.

Following procedures such as liposuction, patients may have swelling, bruising, and discomfort; however, these side effects usually go away in a few weeks as the body heals.

Following a procedure, patients are usually instructed to wear compression garments to reduce swelling and support the newly contoured areas. These garments also help with skin retraction and promote circulation, which improves the final aesthetic result. Patients are also advised to avoid heavy lifting and strenuous activities during the initial phase of recovery to allow the treated areas to heal naturally. The length of recovery time will depend on the extent of treatment, but recovery time from non-surgical options is typically shorter than that from surgical procedures.

Consistent adherence to prescribed medications and skincare regimens, such as maintaining clean and moisturized incision sites, supports healthy tissue recovery and minimizes the risk of complications.

CHAPTER THREE

HOW TO GET READY FOR BODY CONTOURING

PROCESS OF CONSULTATION AND ASSESSMENT

During the initial phases of body contouring, the consultation and assessment process is crucial in determining the best course of action for those who wish to change their bodies. The consultation and assessment process starts with a thorough discussion about the patient's medical history, present state of health, and desired aesthetic outcome. This conversation aids in the creation of a customized treatment plan that is suited to the patient's specific requirements. During the assessment, the practitioner may perform physical examinations and assessments of the areas that need to be treated. Measurements and pictures are used as tools to record the baseline and monitor the patient's progress over time.

A successful body contouring journey begins with patients having a clear understanding of what to expect before, during, and after the procedure. The consultation phase also provides patients with an educational opportunity as they learn about the various body contouring techniques available, their potential benefits, and associated risks. The practitioner, on the other hand, provides expert guidance on realistic outcomes based on the patient's anatomy and skin type. Clear communication and mutual understanding established during this phase lay the groundwork for a successful body contouring journey.

By the time this phase ends, both parties should have a clear understanding and agreement on the treatment plan, improving patient satisfaction and optimizing outcomes. Practitioners also discuss post-procedure care and recovery expectations as part of the consultation and assessment process. This includes outlining potential risks and complications, although they are rare, to ensure patients are well-informed decision-makers.

CANDIDACY AND ELIGIBILITY OF PATIENTS

To guarantee safety and effectiveness, several factors must be evaluated to determine a patient's eligibility and candidacy for body contouring procedures. Those who meet these requirements are usually in good general health, have reasonable expectations for the results, and intend to follow through with a healthy lifestyle after the procedure. These factors may include skin elasticity, BMI (body mass index), and the particular areas that the patient wants to have contoured.

Candidates should not smoke or be willing to give up for a while before and after the procedure, as smoking can impair healing and results. Patients with serious medical conditions, those who are pregnant, or those who are nursing may not be advised to undergo body contouring until they meet specific health criteria.

To ensure that the procedure selected is safe and meets the patient's aesthetic goals, a thorough evaluation of the patient's medical history, including any prior surgeries, allergies, or medications they may be taking, is part of the candidacy assessment. By carefully selecting eligible candidates, practitioners can maximize the likelihood of achieving satisfactory outcomes and minimize potential risks associated with the procedure.

EXPECTATIONS FROM THE PATIENT AND PSYCHOLOGICAL FACTORS

To help patients mentally prepare for their transformation journey, practitioners often assess patients' motivations for undergoing body contouring procedures, ensuring that they have realistic expectations about the results and recovery process. Open discussions about potential risks, limitations, and post-procedure adjustments are essential. Body contouring procedures can have a profound impact on patients' psychological well-being and self-image.

In addition, determining a patient's psychological preparedness entails assessing how they perceive their bodies and whether there are any underlying issues regarding body image dissatisfaction. This assessment aids in customizing the treatment plan to improve not only physical appearance but also general self-esteem and emotional health. Professionals may suggest further assistance, like counseling or support groups, for patients who are significantly experiencing psychological distress associated with their bodies.

To reduce the risk of post-procedure dissatisfaction, practitioners must manage patient expectations by being transparent about the expected outcomes of body contouring procedures, including the likelihood of achieving desired results and potential factors that could influence results. By taking psychological factors into account and aligning patient expectations, practitioners can support patients in making decisions that contribute to a positive body contouring experience.

PRE-PROCEDURE GUIDELINES FOR NUTRITION AND EXERCISE

Body contouring procedures require patients to follow certain dietary and exercise guidelines to maximize results and facilitate a seamless recovery. Patients may be advised to consume a balanced diet high in fruits, vegetables, lean proteins, and whole grains in the weeks preceding the procedure. Hydration is also crucial, as drinking enough water preserves skin elasticity and aids in the body's natural healing processes.

Cardiovascular and strength training are the main types of exercise that are recommended to improve overall fitness levels and muscle tone; however, patients should refrain from intense exercise regimens near the procedure date to minimize the risk of injury and guarantee the best possible recovery results. Moreover, giving up alcohol and smoking can have a positive effect on healing and reduce complications both during and after body contouring procedures.

Patients are advised to discuss any medications or supplements they are currently taking with their healthcare provider to ensure compatibility with the procedure. Complying with these pre-procedure guidelines not only prepares the body physically but also improves the overall success and safety of the body contouring experience. Vitamins C and E are examples of nutritional supplements that may be recommended to support immune function and aid in wound healing.

SELECTING A CLINIC OR QUALIFIED PRACTITIONER

The first step in ensuring a safe and successful body contouring procedure is choosing a qualified practitioner or clinic; patients should thoroughly investigate potential providers, confirming their credentials, experience, and body contouring procedure specialization; memberships in professional organizations and certification by recognized medical boards can attest to a practitioner's commitment to upholding high standards of care and continuing education in aesthetic medicine.

It's important to schedule consultations with multiple providers to compare treatment approaches, discuss expected outcomes, and assess overall comfort and rapport with the practitioner. Patients can also ask questions about the clinic's facilities, safety protocols, and emergency plans during these consultations. Referrals and reviews from previous patients can provide insightful information about the practitioner's reputation and patient satisfaction levels.

Evaluating the clinic's accreditation and compliance with regulations guarantees that the setting satisfies strict health and safety regulations. It is also important to be transparent about procedure costs, including any possible extra fees, to prevent unpleasant surprises later on. Patients can feel secure in their choice of a qualified professional or clinic and concentrate on reaching their desired aesthetic goals with the help of a reliable and trustworthy provider.

CHAPTER FOUR

TECHNIQUES FOR LIPOSUCTION

RECOGNIZING MODERN VS. TRADITIONAL LIPOSUCTION TECHNIQUES

Modern liposuction techniques have largely replaced traditional methods, each with unique advantages and things to keep in mind for body contouring. Traditionally, liposuction has been done by using a cannula, which is a thin tube attached to a vacuum device, to suction out excess fat from specific areas. This method works well for larger fat volumes but may require more downtime and recovery.

On the other hand, modern techniques like tumescent liposuction use a fluid injection to help with fat removal, minimizing blood loss and post-operative discomfort. Another modern technique, laser-assisted liposuction, uses laser energy to liquefy fat before removal, which can result in smoother results and possibly faster healing times.

Selecting between classic and contemporary liposuction techniques frequently comes down to personal taste, health issues, and the particular regions that need to be removed from fat. Knowing these techniques helps patients make decisions based on expectations for recovery and desired results. By speaking with a licensed cosmetic surgeon, patients can determine which technique best suits their medical history and body contouring objectives, guaranteeing a safe and efficient procedure catered to their needs.

OPTIONS FOR ANESTHESIA AND THEIR IMPACTS

Depending on the degree of fat removal and the patient's tolerance level, several options for anesthesia can be chosen. For minor liposuction procedures, for example, local anesthesia is often used to numb the targeted area while the patient is awake. This option allows for a quicker recovery and lower risks associated with general anesthesia. For more extensive procedures, like large-volume liposuction or multiple areas of treatment, general anesthesia may be recommended to ensure patient comfort throughout the surgery.

Patients and surgeons alike must be aware of the effects of each anesthesia option to minimize risks and maximize procedural outcomes. Local anesthesia presents benefits like shorter recovery times and fewer systemic side effects in contrast to general anesthesia, which can involve longer recovery times and possible risks related to deeper sedation

COMPREHENSIVE PROCESS OVERVIEW

A thin, hollow tube called a cannula is inserted through these incisions and used to loosen excess fat deposits. In traditional liposuction, the cannula is connected to a vacuum device that suctions out the fat; however, modern techniques may involve additional steps like laser energy or tumescent fluid injection to facilitate fat removal and enhance skin tightening. The liposuction procedure typically starts with the administration of anesthesia, either local or general, to ensure patient comfort throughout the surgery.

Following fat removal, the incisions are usually closed with sutures or allowed to heal naturally, depending on the surgeon's preference and the extent of the procedure. Post-operative care and recovery instructions are provided to ensure optimal healing and long-term results, including wearing compression garments to minimize swelling and support the new body contours. The surgeon carefully contours the treated areas throughout the procedure to achieve symmetrical and natural-looking results, paying close attention to body proportions and patient aesthetic goals.

CONTROLLING COMPLICATIONS AND RISKS

Liposuction, like any surgical procedure, has potential risks and complications that should be carefully managed to ensure patient safety and satisfactory results.

These complications can include uneven fat removal, skin irregularities, or changes in skin sensation; these can be prevented by careful surgical technique and adherence to sterile protocols. Other common risks include infection, bleeding, and adverse reactions to anesthesia.

Patients can minimize risks and promote a smooth recovery process by adhering to post-operative care instructions and attending follow-up appointments. Surgeons may recommend lifestyle modifications, such as maintaining a healthy diet and regular exercise, to sustain long-term results and enhance overall well-being, supporting liposuction's benefits as a transformative body contouring option.

GETTING NATURAL AND SYMMETRICAL OUTCOMES

Surgeons evaluate each patient's unique anatomy and aesthetic preferences before planning the procedure, identifying areas for fat removal and contour refinement.

During surgery, the surgeon carefully removes excess fat while preserving surrounding tissues and ensuring harmonious proportions, enhancing overall body symmetry and balance. The main goal of liposuction procedures is to achieve symmetrical and natural-looking results, which require meticulous attention to detail and an artistic approach to body contouring.

Surgeons can achieve smoother, more natural contours with advanced techniques like power- or ultrasound-assisted liposuction. Post-operative care, such as wearing compression garments and keeping up recommended activity levels, supports the healing process and helps maintain optimal results. Surgeons can monitor progress, address any concerns, and offer guidance on long-term body contouring strategies during routine follow-up appointments.

CHAPTER FIVE

NON-SURGICAL TECHNIQUES FOR BODY CONTOURING

COOLSCULPTING: WHAT TO EXPECT AND HOW IT OPERATES

Cryolipolysis, another name for CoolSculpting, is a non-invasive body contouring method that targets stubborn fat deposits. It works by subjecting fat cells to a temperature that causes them to naturally die, sparing surrounding tissues.

A specialized applicator is applied to the targeted area, like the thighs or abdomen, and patients usually feel cold at first, then numb as the area becomes numb. Treatment times vary depending on the size and number of areas being treated, but typically last 35 to 60 minutes each session.

CoolSculpting is appropriate for people with localized fat deposits who are close to their ideal body weight but struggle with areas that resist diet and exercise.

Patients may experience temporary redness, swelling, or bruising after the session, but these side effects usually resolve within a few days. Results from CoolSculpting become noticeable gradually as the body naturally eliminates the treated fat cells over several weeks. It is crucial to maintain a healthy diet and regular exercise routine to optimize and prolong the results.

RADIOFREQUENCY AND ULTRASOUND DEVICES: WORKING PRINCIPLES

Both non-surgical body contouring techniques—ultrasound and radiofrequency—achieve fat reduction and skin tightening through different mechanisms. Ultrasound devices target and heat fat cells below the skin's surface using focused ultrasound waves, which causes the fat cells to break down and be absorbed by the body.

This process, called ultrasound cavitation, can also stimulate collagen production, which over time leads to firmer, more toned skin.

On the other hand, radiofrequency (RF) devices deliver energy in the form of radiofrequency waves deep into the skin layers. This energy produces heat, which tightens existing collagen fibers and encourages the production of new collagen, improving skin elasticity and diminishing the appearance of cellulite. To maximize results, RF treatments are frequently coupled with ultrasound or other technologies, providing a flexible method of body contouring.

Both ultrasound and radiofrequency (RF) treatments are generally well-tolerated, requiring no downtime and little discomfort. A few weeks between treatments to allow the body to process the fat and collagen remodeling may be needed for best results. These procedures are appropriate for people who want to have firmer skin, reduce cellulite, and improve body contours without going under the knife.

UTILIZING LASER THERAPY TO REDUCE BODY FAT AND TIGHTEN SKIN

Laser devices emit specific wavelengths of light that penetrate the skin and are absorbed by fat cells, disrupting the fat cells' structure and causing them to break down and eventually be eliminated by the body's lymphatic system. Laser treatments can also stimulate collagen production, which improves skin elasticity and reduces sagging. These benefits have revolutionized non-surgical body contouring.

Similar to other non-surgical methods, laser therapy requires multiple sessions spaced weeks apart to achieve gradual fat reduction and skin tightening effects; however, individual factors such as skin type, age, and the initial condition of the targeted area affect the results. The procedure is generally comfortable, with patients reporting a warming sensation as the laser is applied to the skin.

For those seeking a non-invasive method of body contouring, laser therapy is a good option for those with mild to moderate skin laxity and areas of unwanted fat. A qualified practitioner can help determine the best course of action based on each patient's unique goals and expectations.

COMPARING EFFICIENCY AND APPLICABILITY TO VARIOUS BODY SHAPES

When thinking about non-surgical body contouring techniques, it's important to know how the efficacy and suitability of each technique vary depending on the body type and areas of concern. For example, CoolSculpting is a great way to reduce fat locally in areas like the abdomen, flanks, and thighs, and it works best for people whose fat can be pinchable and suctioned into the treatment applicator.

Both ultrasound and radiofrequency devices can be used to treat different body types. Ultrasound is good for larger areas and can target deeper fat layers, so it's good for people with thicker fat deposits. tighten skin, so they're good for people with mild to moderate skin laxity.

Those with localized fat deposits and mild skin laxity can benefit from laser therapy, which combines skin tightening and fat reduction. The exact wavelength and energy levels used, as well as the practitioner's skill in effectively targeting various body areas, will determine how effective the treatment is.

Selecting the best non-surgical body contouring technique requires taking into account each patient's unique body type, treatment objectives, and the professional's recommendation based on experience and knowledge. A one-on-one consultation with a certified provider can help identify the best strategy to accomplish desired results.

COMBINING NON-SURGICAL METHODS TO IMPROVE OUTCOMES

Combining various non-surgical techniques can provide enhanced benefits for those looking for comprehensive body contouring results. For example, combining CoolSculpting with ultrasound or radiofrequency treatments can target skin tightening and fat reduction in complementary ways, allowing for customized treatment plans that address multiple body concerns at once.

Ultrasound cavitation targets deeper fat layers, while radiofrequency devices improve skin elasticity and texture. Combined, these two techniques can enhance fat reduction and skin tightening effects and lead to more noticeable and significant improvements in body contours over time.

Furthermore, by targeting particular areas of fat and addressing concerns related to skin laxity, combining laser therapy with other techniques can further refine results. Laser treatments can be customized to different wavelengths and energy levels to optimize fat reduction and stimulate collagen production.

To ensure safe and effective treatment combinations catered to individual needs, however, it is imperative to speak with an experienced practitioner.

CHAPTER SIX

HEALING AND FOLLOW-UP

QUICK POST-PROCEDURE HEALING ADVICE

Following body contouring procedures, you should prioritize your immediate post-procedure recovery to minimize pain and maximize healing. You should also carefully follow your surgeon's instructions, which usually include wearing compression garments to minimize swelling and support your newly contoured areas; these garments help to minimize bruising and maintain the shape that was achieved during surgery. You should also make sure that you have someone to help you during the first 24 to 48 hours after the procedure, as you may feel drowsy or dizzy from anesthesia.

Your surgeon may prescribe pain medication to help you manage pain and discomfort. It's important to take these medications exactly as prescribed and to avoid activities that could put strain on the treated areas. You should also stay hydrated, avoid alcohol and tobacco products, and walk gently to promote blood circulation and lower your risk of blood clots. Finally, keep an eye out for any signs of infection, such as increased redness, swelling, or drainage, and get in touch with your surgeon right away if you notice any concerning symptoms.

HANDLING PAIN AND SWELLING

After body contouring procedures, discomfort and swelling are common, but there are effective ways to manage these symptoms and encourage healing. One way to significantly reduce swelling after surgery is to elevate the treated areas and allow fluid to drain naturally. During the first few days after surgery, try to keep the affected areas elevated above your heart. This position encourages fluid to drain away from the surgical site, which minimizes swelling and discomfort.

A healthy diet rich in fruits, vegetables, and lean proteins can also help reduce inflammation and promote healing. Finally, drinking plenty of water can help flush out toxins from your body and support overall recovery. Applying cold compresses on occasion can also help reduce swelling and ease discomfort. Use ice packs wrapped in a cloth or a specially designed cooling pad, applying them for about 20 minutes at a time, several times a day. However, avoid applying ice directly to your skin to prevent frostbite.

ADVICE ON NUTRITION AND DIET FOLLOWING PROCEDURE

After body contouring procedures, optimal recovery and long-term results depend on proper nutrition. Your diet should support tissue repair, reduce inflammation, and promote healing. Include foods high in vitamins A and C, which are essential for collagen production and wound healing; high-vitamin foods include oranges, strawberries, spinach, and sweet potatoes. Lean proteins, like chicken, fish, tofu, and legumes, provide the building blocks needed for tissue repair.

Omega-3 fatty acids—found in fish like salmon and flaxseeds—help lower inflammation and increase skin elasticity. Steer clear of processed foods, high amounts of salt and sugary snacks; instead, choose whole grains like brown rice and quinoa, which offer sustained energy and vital nutrients.

Maintain stable blood sugar levels throughout the day to aid in your body's healing process. Speaking with a nutritionist or your surgeon can help customize a post-operative diet plan that suits your unique needs.

EXTENDED CARE TO SUSTAIN OUTCOMES

A commitment to long-term care and healthy lifestyle practices is necessary to maintain the results of your body contouring procedure. Exercise is essential for toning and maintaining muscle tone, which can enhance the contours achieved through surgery. Include both strength training exercises specifically targeted at the treated areas and cardiovascular exercises such as walking or cycling. This balanced approach helps burn calories, reduce fat deposits, and improve overall body shape.

Exercise alone won't preserve your results; fluctuations in weight can affect how your contours look; drink lots of water throughout the day to stay hydrated, as this promotes skin elasticity and general health; and lastly, schedule follow-up visits with your surgeon as advised to track your progress and promptly address any concerns. By putting these long-term care practices first, you can reap the benefits of your body contouring procedure for years to come.

TRACKING RECOVERY AND IDENTIFYING RED FLAGS

Keeping a close eye on your incision sites for signs of infection, such as increasing redness, warmth, or drainage, is essential for ensuring optimal recovery and spotting any potential warning signs after body contouring procedures. If you notice any unusual or persistent symptoms, like severe pain that does not improve with prescribed medications, fever, or excessive swelling, get in touch with your surgeon right away for further evaluation.

Follow your surgeon's post-operative instructions carefully, including showing up for scheduled follow-up appointments, so that your surgeon can assess your healing progress, watch for any potential complications, and make recommendations for ongoing care. By being proactive and mindful of your body's needs, you can promote a smooth recovery and get the best results from your body contouring procedure. Pay attention to your body's signals and be open and honest with your healthcare provider about any concerns you may have.

CHAPTER SEVEN

HAZARDS AND DIFFICULTIES

TYPICAL ADVERSE REACTIONS FOLLOWING BODY CONTOURING

Patients should be aware that body contouring procedures, whether surgical or non-surgical, can have several common side effects, which include swelling, bruising, and temporary discomfort at the treatment site. Pain is also common, but usually manageable with prescribed medications. Patients may also experience numbness or tingling, particularly in the areas where skin tightening or fat removal has occurred. Skin irregularities, such as dimpling or uneven contours, can also occur but usually go away over time as the body heals and adapts to the new shape.

Following body contouring, patients should anticipate some limitations in their daily activities and mobility. Sustaining appropriate hydration and nutrition can aid in the healing process, promoting faster healing and lessening the severity of side effects. Frequent follow-up visits with the healthcare team allow for monitoring of progress and early detection of any potential complications. Patients should follow the post-operative care instructions provided by the surgeon or healthcare provider to facilitate optimal healing and minimize these side effects.

Patients can better prepare themselves for the physical and psychological aftermath of body contouring procedures by being aware of these common side effects. Patients who are proactive in managing these effects can navigate their recovery period more comfortably and feel more confident about the results of their procedure.

RARE BUT DANGEROUS SIDE EFFECTS INCLUDE NERVE DAMAGE, INFECTION, AND SCARRING

Body contouring procedures, although rare, carry the potential risk of serious complications that patients should be aware of.

Nerve damage, though rare, can result in temporary or permanent numbness, altered sensation, or muscle weakness in the treated area. Surgeons take precautions to minimize these risks, but patients should be vigilant in reporting any unusual symptoms post-operatively. Infections can occur despite strict adherence to hygiene protocols, leading to redness, swelling, and increased pain at the surgical site. Patients should seek prompt medical attention if signs of infection develop.

Surgery will always leave scars, but how severe they are will depend on the technique employed and each patient's healing response. Less invasive liposuction or laser-assisted procedures are examples of techniques that try to minimize visible scars and encourage a more seamless recovery. Patients who are worried about scars should talk to their surgeon about scar management options before the procedure to ensure proper post-operative care.

Knowing about these uncommon but potentially dangerous side effects highlights the significance of selecting a board-certified surgeon and carefully adhering to pre-and post-operative instructions. Clear lines of communication with medical professionals enable prompt action in the event of complications, guaranteeing the best possible safety and results for patients having body contouring procedures.

RECOGNIZING THE ROLE OF THE PATIENT IN REDUCING RISKS

Patients who follow pre-operative instructions, such as refraining from certain medications, fasting before surgery, and quitting smoking, significantly reduce the risk of complications during and after the procedure. Patients also play a critical role in minimizing risks associated with body contouring procedures by actively participating in their recovery. Previous surgeries, allergies, and medications must be disclosed to the healthcare team before surgery.

Patients should closely monitor any signs of infection, excessive bleeding, or unusual symptoms and promptly report them to the healthcare provider. Upholding a healthy lifestyle with balanced nutrition and regular physical activity supports the body's healing process and enhances the longevity of results achieved through body contouring. Patients should adhere to all post-operative care instructions meticulously during recovery, including wound care, activity restrictions, and attending scheduled follow-up appointments.

Patients who actively participate in their care and partner with their healthcare team are much more likely to achieve optimal aesthetic results safely and effectively after body contouring procedures. Taking personal responsibility for minimizing risks not only promotes a smoother recovery but also increases overall satisfaction with the results.

ETHICAL AND LEGAL ASPECTS OF PATIENT CONSENT

Informed consent entails ensuring that patients understand the nature of the procedure, potential risks and benefits, alternative treatments, and expected outcomes. It also involves disclosing information about the surgeon's qualifications, facility accreditation, and expected recovery process to enable patients to make well-informed decisions. Obtaining informed consent from patients before body contouring procedures involves ethical and legal considerations that healthcare providers must carefully navigate.

Healthcare providers must effectively communicate with patients, answering their questions and concerns transparently and understandably. Carefully documenting the informed consent process in the patient's medical record demonstrates compliance with legal standards and ethical principles governing patient care. Ethical considerations in informed consent emphasize patient autonomy, respect for individual values, and the right to withdraw consent at any time before or during the procedure.

Failing to obtain valid informed consent can result in legal consequences, underscoring the significance of clear communication, documentation, and adherence to established protocols in patient care. Legal implications of informed consent require healthcare providers to comply with state and federal regulations governing medical practice, including those related to patient rights, privacy, and professional liability.

Managing the complexity of informed consent guarantees that patients having body contouring operations are protected by ethical and legal norms in healthcare practice, fully informed, and empowered to make decisions that are in line with their personal preferences and health goals.

MANAGING EXPECTATIONS AND RESOLVING PATIENT CONCERNS

Successful body contouring procedures require proactive management of patient expectations and concerns as well as effective communication. Patients may have different expectations about the procedure's potential risks, recovery times, and outcomes.

Healthcare providers are critical in addressing these concerns through thorough pre-operative consultations, realistic goal-setting, and explanation of potential limitations based on individual anatomy and health status.

Setting realistic goals helps align patient expectations with the anticipated results of body contouring procedures, improving overall satisfaction and lowering the likelihood of disappointment post-operatively. Healthcare providers should encourage open dialogue, actively listen to patient concerns, and provide empathetic support throughout the treatment journey. Managing patient expectations involves providing realistic assessments of achievable outcomes and discussing potential complications openly and transparently.

The psychological and emotional aspects of body image and self-esteem must also be addressed to manage patient expectations. Constant communication and individualized care helps to establish rapport and trust between patients and healthcare providers, which fosters a collaborative approach to safely and effectively achieving desired aesthetic outcomes. Supporting patients in understanding the transformative but gradual nature of aesthetic changes and offering reassurance during the recovery period promote positive outcomes and patient satisfaction.

CHAPTER EIGHT

ACHIEVING RESULTS THAT SEEM NATURAL

BODY CONTOURING ARTISTRY: SCULPTING & SCULPTING BIOLOGICAL CURVES

Professionals use advanced sculpting tools and techniques tailored to individual body shapes, emphasizing harmony and balance. By focusing on enhancing natural curves rather than drastic changes, practitioners achieve results that complement the patient's physique. The process of body contouring involves meticulous planning to ensure that contours appear smooth and proportionate, enhancing the overall aesthetic appeal. Overall, body contouring is an art form that aims to enhance natural body curves through strategic fat removal and sculpting techniques.

To achieve a smooth transition between treated and untreated areas for a seamless appearance, techniques like liposuction and fat grafting are frequently used to refine body contours. While fat grafting redistributes fat to areas that may benefit from enhancement, such as the buttocks or breasts, liposuction targets localized fat deposits. The artistry lies in achieving a sculpted look that appears natural, respecting the body's inherent proportions and contours. Practitioners frequently use 3D imaging and simulations to visualize potential outcomes, ensuring that the desired aesthetic goals are realistically aligned with expectations.

Expertise in both the medical and artistic domains is necessary to achieve natural-looking body contours. Surgeons evaluate each patient's unique anatomy and aesthetic objectives to develop a customized contouring plan. This entails knowing how various body areas interact and making sure that enhancements add to rather than take away from natural beauty. By emphasizing artistry in body contouring, practitioners can achieve results that boost confidence and overall satisfaction.

PREVENTING OVERCORRECTION AND IMPRACTICAL ASPIRATIONS

Successful body contouring involves avoiding overcorrection and controlling patient expectations. Overcorrection is when too much fat is removed or added, leading to unnatural or disproportionate results. Skilled practitioners prioritize subtle enhancements that complement the body's natural contours, avoiding excessive alterations that may result in dissatisfaction. Surgeons ensure that patients understand what is realistically achievable through thorough consultation and realistic goal-setting. This includes discussing limitations and potential outcomes based on individual anatomy and medical considerations.

Establishing realistic expectations and helping patients visualize possible changes to their bodies are the first steps in managing unrealistic expectations. Practitioners educate and inform patients about the limitations of body contouring procedures and show them before-and-after photos that demonstrate achievable results. By showcasing real patient outcomes, practitioners build trust and make sure that patients are aware of what to expect after the procedure. They also talk about potential follow-up procedures or adjustments that may be necessary to optimize results over time.

The attainment of favorable results in body contouring is contingent upon the balancing of patient desires and surgical expertise. Surgeons stress the significance of gradual enhancements that maintain the body's natural contours, refraining from drastic modifications that may jeopardize aesthetic harmony.

By emphasizing patient education and realistic expectations, they reduce the likelihood of patient dissatisfaction and guarantee that results are in line with each patient's objectives. This strategy not only improves physical appearance but also fosters confidence and satisfaction in achieving results that look natural.

UTILIZING BEFORE-AND-AFTER IMAGES AS ACCURATE REFERENCES

During consultations, surgeons use before-and-after photos to show potential improvements and discuss realistic expectations, stressing the importance of individual variability in outcomes. These images showcase actual patient results, demonstrating the transformative effects of contouring procedures like fat grafting or liposuction. Patients gain insight into what can be achieved and how their bodies may change after the procedure from looking at these photos.

The ability of patients to visually evaluate the efficacy of various procedures and comprehend how particular treatments can enhance their natural contours is demonstrated by before-and-after photos, which showcase improvements in body shape and proportion. Carefully chosen to represent a range of outcomes, these images assist patients in visualizing potential changes and informing decisions about their care. Surgeons use these visuals to customize treatment plans to each patient's unique anatomy and aesthetic goals, ensuring personalized and satisfying results.

Before-and-after photos are a visual communication tool that surgeons use to educate patients about the advantages and limitations of body contouring, emphasizing realistic expectations and potential variations in outcomes. This visual communication tool increases patient satisfaction and confidence in decision-making, paving the way for successful body contouring experiences. Patients are encouraged to ask questions and express their preferences based on visual evidence, fostering a collaborative approach to treatment planning.

PATIENT EDUCATION REGARDING REASONABLE EXPECTATIONS FOR RESULTS

Patient education is essential to body contouring, especially when it comes to controlling expectations about realistic results. Surgeons educate patients about the potential and constraints of contouring procedures, stressing the individual variability in results. They also help patients understand how factors like skin elasticity, fat distribution, and anatomical considerations affect post-procedural outcomes. By providing informed information, practitioners help patients set reasonable expectations and feel empowered to make decisions about their aesthetic goals.

Patient satisfaction is contingent upon an understanding of the variability of body contouring outcomes. Surgeons clarify that although procedures such as liposuction or fat grafting can improve body contours, individual factors, including age, skin quality, and general health, can affect how the body responds to treatment. Surgeons ensure that patients receive comprehensive information and are aware of potential changes in body shape and contour over time.

Prioritizing patient education allows surgeons to empower patients to make informed decisions about their aesthetic goals and achieve satisfying, long-lasting results. They also discuss the recovery process and potential follow-up care needed to optimize results. Surgeons outline realistic timelines for recovery and emphasize the importance of post-operative instructions to promote healing and minimize complications. Patients feel prepared and confident for their body contouring journey, knowing what to expect at each stage of treatment.

PROCEDURES FOR FOLLOW-UP AND ANY ADJUSTMENTS

A proactive approach to body contouring ensures that patients maintain satisfaction with their results and achieve the desired aesthetic goals. While initial procedures such as liposuction or fat grafting can create significant improvements, refinement may be necessary to address any residual concerns or changes in body shape. Surgeons schedule follow-up appointments to assess healing progress, evaluate outcomes, and discuss any additional treatments that may enhance results.

Follow-up procedures allow surgeons to monitor recovery and offer ongoing support as patients transition into enjoying their enhanced physique. Adjustments may involve small touch-ups or complementary procedures designed to fine-tune results and address specific areas of concern. Surgeons collaborate closely with patients to identify areas for improvement and customize treatment plans accordingly. This collaborative approach fosters trust and ensures that patient expectations are met, promoting long-term satisfaction with body contouring outcomes.

A surgeon's commitment to patient care and satisfaction is demonstrated by the follow-up procedures and adjustments that they provide. These sessions offer patients the chance to discuss any concerns they may have following surgery, refine their results, and make sure they get the most out of their body contouring experience. This all-encompassing approach to care not only improves aesthetic outcomes but also strengthens the relationship between the patient and the surgeon, which is built on trust, openness, and personalized attention. Follow-up procedures are an essential part of successful body contouring journeys because they help patients maintain confidence and satisfaction with their improved appearance.

CHAPTER NINE

FINANCIAL PLANNING AND COST CONSIDERATIONS

RECOGNIZING BODY CONTOURING COST FACTORS

The cost of body contouring procedures can vary greatly depending on several important factors. Firstly, the type of procedure selected is a major cost factor; due to the equipment and complexity of surgical procedures like liposuction, the cost of these procedures is usually higher than that of non-surgical options like CoolSculpting. Secondly, the extent of treatment required directly affects pricing; larger areas or multiple areas require more time and resources from the provider, which drives up costs.

Second, location can have a big influence on costs. In general, urban areas have higher overhead for clinics and surgeons, which means procedure costs are higher there than in rural or suburban areas. In addition, pricing is also influenced by the surgeon's reputation and experience. Highly experienced surgeons who have a proven track record of success often charge premium fees for their services.

Last but not least, extra expenses like anesthesia, facility fees, and post-operative care must be included in the total cost of body contouring. Anesthesia costs can change depending on the procedure's complexity and length, and facility fees pay for the use of recovery rooms and operating rooms. Post-operative care costs include prescription drugs, compression garments, and follow-up visits, all of which are necessary to ensure optimal healing and results.

CHOICES FOR FINANCING AND INSURANCE PROTECTION

Understanding financing options and insurance coverage is crucial for anyone thinking about getting body contouring procedures done. Most body contouring techniques are considered elective cosmetic procedures, meaning they are not covered by health insurance plans because they are deemed cosmetic rather than medically necessary. However, there may be some exceptions if the procedure is intended to treat a medical condition, such as excess skin following significant weight loss.

Patients can choose payment plans that fit their budget, spreading out the cost of body contouring over time rather than paying upfront. Many cosmetic surgery practices offer payment plans or financing options to help patients manage the cost of treatment. These plans often involve third-party financing companies that specialize in medical loans with flexible repayment terms.

Before committing to a plan, patients should carefully consider their financing options and compare interest rates, fees, and repayment schedules. Moreover, some practices provide additional financial incentives to patients by offering discounts for paying in full upfront or for multiple procedures completed at the same time.

COMPARING VALUE AND PRICE IN VARIOUS PROCESSES

Making an informed decision when weighing body contouring procedures requires weighing the value vs. price. Value includes both the procedure's cost and the anticipated results, such as improved confidence and aesthetic improvements. The value of various procedures varies depending on the goals and expectations of the individual.

Surgical procedures like abdominoplasty (tummy tuck) or body lift surgery generally have higher initial costs but may provide more dramatic and long-lasting results in a single procedure.

Non-surgical procedures like laser fat removal or radiofrequency treatments may offer lower upfront costs and minimal downtime compared to surgical options. However, the results may require multiple sessions to achieve desired outcomes, potentially increasing overall costs over time.

Determining the worth of each procedure entails weighing variables like recovery time, possible risks, and anticipated duration of results.

Speaking with a board-certified plastic surgeon can offer insightful advice about which procedure best suits individual objectives and financial constraints, guaranteeing that the body contouring investment produces results that meet expectations.

SETTING UP A BUDGET FOR SEVERAL PROCEDURES OR FOLLOW-UP VISITS

Careful financial planning is necessary when budgeting for multiple body contouring procedures or follow-up sessions. For patients undergoing comprehensive transformation, like post-bariatric body contouring, sequential procedures targeting different areas of concern should be accounted for. Setting priorities for procedures based on patient goals and surgeon recommendations can help control costs while achieving desired outcomes over time.

Budgeting for follow-up sessions is also necessary to guarantee the best possible healing and maintenance of results. These sessions provide continuity of care and improve overall satisfaction with the body contouring journey. Additional treatments for contour refinement, scar management, or adjustments based on healing progress and aesthetic goals may be included in follow-up sessions.

Patients seeking extensive body contouring transformations can save money by budgeting carefully and prioritizing treatments based on individual needs.

Patients can achieve their desired body contours within their financial means by discussing comprehensive treatment plans with their surgeon, including anticipated costs for multiple procedures and follow-up sessions. Some practices offer package deals or discounts for bundled procedures.

UNDERSTANDING PAYMENT PLANS AND BARGAINING FOR A BETTER PRICE

Patients can often negotiate package pricing for multiple procedures or receive discounts for paying in advance. It's helpful to ask about promotional offers or seasonal specials that clinics may offer to attract new patients or encourage loyalty among existing clients.

Understanding payment plans and negotiating pricing are crucial aspects of managing costs associated with body contouring procedures.

Patients should compare payment plans, taking into account factors like interest rates, repayment terms, and penalties for late payments, to select the most appropriate option for their financial situation. Many practices offer flexible payment options, such as zero-interest financing for a specified period or low-interest medical loans through partnering financial institutions. Understanding payment plans involves carefully reading terms and conditions.

Patients can make informed decisions that are in line with their desired aesthetic outcomes and budgetary constraints by proactively exploring pricing options and payment plans. Surgeons and clinic staff are often willing to work with patients to accommodate their financial needs while ensuring access to high-quality body contouring services. Patients can facilitate discussions on customized payment plans or potential discounts by being transparent about their financial goals and limitations with the cosmetic surgery practice.

CHAPTER TEN

SELECTING THE CORRECT CLINIC AND PROVIDER

EXAMINING EXPERIENCE AND CERTIFICATIONS

It's important to look for additional certifications or memberships in professional organizations related to body contouring, such as the American Society of Plastic Surgeons or the American Academy of Dermatology, as these affiliations often indicate ongoing education and adherence to ethical standards. When researching credentials and experience for body contouring procedures, it's important to prioritize qualifications that ensure safety and quality outcomes. Start by confirming that the provider is board-certified in plastic surgery or dermatology, as this signifies specialized training and adherence to high standards of practice.

When choosing a provider, experience is also very important. Find out how long the provider has been doing body contouring procedures and if they specialize in the techniques you're interested in, like abdominoplasty, liposuction, or non-surgical options like CoolSculpting. You can also find out how many procedures the provider performs annually and how satisfied their patients are. You can also find out if the provider has completed any fellowships or specialized training in aesthetic procedures to confirm their experience.

In addition, examine prior patient before-and-after pictures to evaluate the provider's track record of meeting your aesthetic objectives. This visual proof can reveal information about the provider's level of expertise and capacity to customize treatments for each patient. By carefully examining the credentials and experience of the provider, you can feel more assured about choosing one who places a high priority on safety, knowledge, and reaching the best possible body contouring outcomes.

PATIENT TESTIMONIALS AND REVIEWS: WHAT TO LOOK FOR

Patient testimonials and reviews provide insightful firsthand information about the experience and results of body contouring procedures. When reading reviews, give priority to those that describe the full patient journey, from initial consultation to post-operative care. Look for a pattern of positive comments about the provider's bedside manner, communication skills, and responsiveness to concerns. Take note of any mentions of results, and consider whether they line up with your goals for body contouring.

Look for reviews that address particular procedures you are thinking about, like body lifts or liposuction; these in-depth narratives can give you a realistic expectation of recovery times, degree of discomfort, and overall satisfaction with the result. You should also take into consideration reviews that address any unexpected outcomes or complications; this openness can help you emotionally and psychologically prepare for the procedure.

In the end, patient reviews and testimonials are a great way to learn about the possible advantages and difficulties of body contouring procedures. Testimonials frequently highlight personal transformations and improvements in self-confidence, offering qualitative insights beyond clinical outcomes.

EXAMINING CLINICS AND ESTABLISHING STANDARDS FOR FACILITIES

Attending clinics in person is a crucial first step in evaluating facility standards for body contouring procedures.

When you arrive, check the state of the treatment rooms and reception area. A clean and orderly space not only conveys professionalism but also lowers the risk of infection and guarantees a comfortable experience for patients. Notice the atmosphere in general and if it matches your expectations for a secure and welcoming medical setting.

When you visit, find out if the clinic is accredited by the Joint Commission or the Accreditation Association for Ambulatory Health Care (AAC). This shows that the clinic complies with strict guidelines regarding emergency planning, equipment sterilization, and patient safety. You should also find out about the credentials and experience of the clinical staff, which includes the nurses and anesthesiologists who will be performing your procedure.

Examine the clinic's technology and equipment, especially the body contouring procedures you are considering. State-of-the-art technology can improve procedural accuracy and reduce recovery times. Find out if the clinic offers post-operative care resources and facilities, like overnight stays or outpatient recovery areas, to guarantee all-encompassing assistance during your recuperation.

You may make an educated selection based on the standard of care and setting by visiting clinics and evaluating facility standards directly. This proactive approach gives you peace of mind regarding the provider's dedication to patient safety and comfort.

WHAT TO ASK IN A CONSULTATION

Asking focused questions can help you feel more in control of your decision-making during your consultation for body contouring procedures. Begin by going over the specific available procedure options, including both surgical and non-surgical approaches, and how each fits with your medical history and aesthetic goals. Find out about the procedure's expected results, recovery times, and potential risks to make sure you have reasonable expectations.

Talk about the anesthesia options available and the credentials of the anesthesiologist who will administer it during your procedure. Inquire about the provider's experience with cases similar to yours and their success rates in achieving desired outcomes. Ask to see before-and-after photos of patients with body types and concerns similar to yours, as visual evidence can illustrate the provider's expertise and artistic approach to body contouring.

Make sure you understand the cost of the procedure, including any potential additional fees for anesthesia, facility use, or post-operative care. Find out about financing options or payment plans if necessary to ensure financial preparedness. Find out about the recovery timeline and when you can expect to resume normal activities, including exercise and work.

Finally, follow your gut during the consultation. Determine how at ease you are with the provider's manner, communication style, and willingness to address your concerns.

USING YOUR GUT SENTIMENT AND MAKING WELL-INFORMED CHOICES

A genuine connection and mutual understanding can foster trust and confidence in the healthcare professional's ability to deliver satisfactory results. During and after the consultation, consider how comfortable you were with the provider, the clinic environment, and the proposed treatment plan. Take into account how well your questions were answered and whether the provider listened to your concerns and goals.

Examine the data you've gathered from looking up credentials, reading patient testimonials, going to clinics, and asking questions during consultations. Consider any concerns or red flags that come up during this process and be honest with the provider about them. Being transparent and communicating openly is crucial to feeling empowered and fully informed to make decisions that suit your priorities and expectations.

Seek advice from family members or trusted friends who can guide you through the decision-making process. If you are unsure about the suggested course of treatment or the provider, get a second opinion.

CHAPTER ELEVEN

TRENDS IN BODY CONTOURING IN THE FUTURE

TECHNOLOGICAL AND TECHNIQUE INNOVATIONS

The field of body contouring has undergone a revolution with the introduction of more precise and minimally invasive procedures for achieving desired body shapes. Two noteworthy innovations in this regard are the increasing popularity of non-surgical options such as cryolipolysis and ultrasound treatments, which target and reduce fat cells without the need for surgery and are popular with patients who want minimal downtime and natural-looking results. Another innovation is the development of laser-assisted liposuction, which uses laser energy to liquefy fat deposits before removal, improving precision and stimulating collagen production.

Another technological advance is robotic-assisted body contouring, which uses robotic arms to perform liposuction with improved precision and less trauma to surrounding tissues, resulting in more predictable results and faster recovery times.3D imaging technology has also become essential to treatment planning, allowing surgeons to plan procedures according to individual anatomy and simulate results. These developments highlight a trend toward individualized treatments that accommodate patient preferences and guarantee safer, more effective outcomes.

With ongoing research into stem cell therapy and tissue engineering, which aim to improve graft survival rates and integrate with natural tissues seamlessly, the future of body contouring appears bright. When combined with developments in virtual reality for patient education and outcome visualization, the field of body contouring is poised to provide even more customized and satisfying results, catering to the various needs of patients seeking body sculpting solutions.

PREFERENCE TRENDS THAT ARE NOT YET ESTABLISHING

There has been a noticeable shift in patient preferences in recent years toward less invasive procedures and natural-looking results in body contouring; patients are choosing treatments that accentuate their natural contours without making drastic changes, indicating a desire for subtle improvements that complement their overall appearance.

This trend has prompted advancements in techniques like fat transfer, which involves purifying and re-using fat harvested from one area to augment other areas, such as the buttocks or breasts, providing a more comprehensive approach to body sculpting.

Additionally, there is a growing need for treatment plans that are customized to each patient's unique body type and aesthetic goals. In response, clinics are providing thorough consultations and simulating procedures using advanced imaging technologies so that patients know exactly what to expect after the procedure. Patient safety and comfort are still the top priorities, which has led to the adoption of methods like sedation and local anesthesia that reduce risks and improve recovery times.

Understanding patient preferences is important for practitioners who aim to provide patient-centered care and achieve high levels of satisfaction. Cultural influences also play a significant role in shaping patient preferences.

For example, different regions express different ideals of beauty and body image. In some cultures, curvier silhouettes are favored, which leads to increased interest in procedures that enhance natural curves through techniques like Brazilian butt lifts. As these trends evolve, the body contouring field continues to adapt, offering tailored solutions that respect cultural diversity while delivering safe and effective outcomes.

FORECASTS FOR INCREASES IN SAFETY AND EFFICACY

With continued research and technological advancements, body contouring is expected to undergo significant safety and efficacy advancements. Safer anesthesia protocols and techniques that ensure patient comfort and shorten recovery times are one promising area of development. Surgical instruments and techniques that improve precision and reduce trauma to surrounding tissues also bode well for faster healing and more predictable results.

Personalized recovery plans and remote monitoring technologies are two examples of how advances in post-operative care are improving patient experiences and lowering complications. Additionally, the integration of artificial intelligence (AI) and machine learning into treatment planning is transforming the way procedures are carried out. AI algorithms can analyze patient data and imaging scans to optimize surgical plans, ensuring the highest level of accuracy and customization.

This predictive modeling not only enhances safety but also improves efficacy by tailoring treatments to individual anatomies and desired outcomes.

The field of body contouring is expected to undergo continuous improvement due to the ongoing evolution of regulatory standards and guidelines on a global scale, which ensure that practitioners follow strict safety protocols and uphold high standards of care. Patients can anticipate safer procedures, quicker recoveries, and more satisfying aesthetic outcomes as these innovations emerge, ushering in a new era in cosmetic surgery.

INTERNATIONAL VIEWS AND CULTURAL AFFECTS

Diverse ideals of beauty and aesthetic preferences are reflected in the wide range of body contouring practices and preferences that are found across different regions and cultures. In Western countries, for example, there is often a focus on achieving an athletic and toned physique, which drives demand for procedures like high-definition liposuction and abdominal etching. These procedures aim to sculpt the body to emphasize muscle definition and create a chiseled appearance, which is in line with cultural preferences for fitness and body positivity.

On the other hand, procedures like hip enhancement and buttock augmentation are common in areas where curvier silhouettes are traditionally valued. These regions also value natural curves and proportions, so procedures like fat transfer—where fat is harvested from one area and injected into the buttocks or hips—cater to these preferences by reflecting cultural ideals of beauty while also empowering patients to achieve their desired aesthetic goals while maintaining authenticity and cultural identity.

Furthermore, the world's views on body contouring are shaped by developments in technology and the availability of novel treatments. Nations possessing highly developed healthcare systems and regulatory environments are frequently at the forefront of implementing novel approaches and guaranteeing optimal safety and effectiveness. Conversely, developing nations may witness a sharp increase in the demand for cosmetic procedures due to improved accessibility and shifting societal perceptions of beauty.

Ultimately, to provide culturally sensitive and effective care, practitioners must have a thorough understanding of global perspectives and cultural influences. By honoring various ideals of beauty and customizing treatments to each patient's preferences, practitioners can make sure that body contouring procedures improve patient confidence and well-being in a variety of cultural contexts.

OPPORTUNITIES FOR PROFESSIONAL DEVELOPMENT AND CONTINUING EDUCATION

Body contouring is a dynamic and ever-evolving field that provides a wealth of opportunities for professional development and ongoing education.

Specialized training programs and workshops allow practitioners to stay up to date on the latest technological and procedural advancements. By giving practitioners hands-on experience with new tools and procedures, these educational opportunities equip practitioners with the skills and knowledge necessary to deliver superior patient outcomes.

Furthermore, certifications and credentials in cosmetic surgery and body sculpting validate expertise and reassure patients of practitioner qualifications. Professional organizations and societies also play a crucial role in fostering collaboration and knowledge sharing among practitioners. Membership in these organizations offers access to resources like research publications, clinical guidelines, and networking events that promote best practices and innovation in body contouring.

Combining medical knowledge with holistic approaches to health and wellness, practitioners can address both aesthetic goals and underlying health considerations, promoting long-term patient satisfaction and well-being. As the field develops further, continuing professional development guarantees that practitioners stay at the forefront of advancements, delivering safe, effective, and creative body contouring solutions. The integration of multidisciplinary approaches, including collaborations with nutritionists, fitness experts, and dermatologists, enhances comprehensive patient care and expands treatment options.

CHAPTER TWELVE

FAQS & FREQUENTLY ASKED QUESTIONS

THE DANGERS OF BODY CONTOURING

Surgical and non-surgical body contouring procedures have inherent risks that patients should be aware of. Anesthesia is a risk factor for surgical procedures like liposuction; it can also cause allergic reactions or adverse effects on the respiratory system. Surgical procedures also carry the risk of infection at the incision sites, though this is reduced by the use of sterile techniques.

Temporary side effects are possible with non-surgical procedures like cryolipolysis (cool sculpting), such as redness, bruising, or numbness in the treated areas, but these usually go away on their own.

Understanding these risks is crucial, and consulting with a qualified cosmetic surgeon can help mitigate them through proper patient selection and technique.

Additionally, both surgical and non-surgical procedures may result in uneven fat removal or irregularities in the contour that may require additional corrective treatments. Skin laxity is another concern, especially in patients with poor skin elasticity, as it may not fully retract after fat reduction, leading to loose or sagging skin.

TIME FRAME FOR BODY CONTOURING OUTCOMES

The durability of body contouring results varies depending on the procedure and individual factors. Non-surgical treatments like radiofrequency or laser therapy can also produce long-lasting results by reducing fat cell volume, though multiple sessions may be necessary for optimal outcomes.

Surgical methods like liposuction typically provide permanent fat removal in treated areas, as fat cells are physically extracted. However, maintaining results requires a healthy lifestyle to prevent new fat accumulation.

Genetics, lifestyle choices, and general health all play a role in longevity. Weight changes can have an impact on outcomes, particularly if there is a noticeable increase in weight following treatment. To maximize and sustain results, patients must adhere to the post-procedure instructions given by their cosmetic surgeon. Frequent follow-up appointments can also help track progress and promptly address any concerns.

INTEGRATING OTHER SURGERY WITH BODY CONTOURING

To achieve comprehensive aesthetic goals, it is common to combine body contouring procedures with other cosmetic surgeries. For example, liposuction and abdominoplasty (tummy tuck) can be used together to address excess skin and muscle laxity in addition to fat removal. This combined approach allows for enhanced body sculpting and contour refinement in targeted areas, resulting in more dramatic and satisfying overall results.

Nonetheless, combining procedures adds to the complexity of the surgery and lengthens the recovery period, so it's critical to talk about expectations, risks, and goals with a board-certified plastic surgeon. They can suggest the best course of action based on each patient's unique anatomy and desired results. Thorough pre-operative evaluations and post-operative care are also necessary to guarantee safety and maximize cosmetic results for patients having combined surgeries.

EXPECTATIONS FOR THE RECOVERING PERIOD

Compression garments may be recommended to minimize swelling and support healing in treated areas. The recovery period after body contouring procedures varies depending on the type and extent of treatment. Generally, surgical methods require more downtime compared to non-surgical options. Patients undergoing abdominoplasty or liposuction should expect initial discomfort, swelling, and bruising, which typically subside within a few weeks.

To achieve the best possible outcome and a smooth recovery, patients should carefully follow post-operative instructions, including wound care and activity restrictions. Patients should plan for adequate rest and avoid strenuous activities during the initial healing phase, gradually returning to normal activities as advised by their surgeon. Non-surgical treatments often involve minimal downtime, with mild side effects like temporary numbness or redness resolving within days to weeks.

SELECTING BETWEEN NON-SURGICAL AND SURGICAL CHOICES

Surgical procedures such as liposuction offer more immediate and dramatic results in terms of fat reduction by physically removing fat cells from targeted areas; this approach is ideal for patients seeking significant body sculpting or those with stubborn fat deposits resistant to diet and exercise. Ultimately, the choice between surgical and non-surgical body contouring options depends on individual goals, preferences, and medical considerations.

With minimal discomfort and downtime, non-surgical techniques like laser therapy, cryolipolysis, or radiofrequency treatments offer gradual body contouring and fat reduction through targeted energy delivery to fat cells. This makes them ideal for people with busy schedules or mild to moderate fat concerns, but results may be subtler than with surgery and may require multiple sessions to achieve desired results.

To determine candidacy for both surgical and non-surgical options based on individual anatomy, medical history, and aesthetic goals, patients must consult with a qualified cosmetic surgeon. They can offer customized recommendations and discuss expected outcomes, risks, and recovery considerations to help patients make well-informed decisions about body contouring treatments.